Living with Early Onset Dementia:

Understanding, Managing, and Thriving

I0490782

Lisa Head

Understanding, Managing and Thriving

Living with Early Onset Dementia

Understanding, Managing and Thriving

DEDICATION

This book is dedicated to all those that live with Early Onset Dementia, their families and their caregivers.

Understanding, Managing and Thriving

CONTENTS

Understanding, Managing and Thriving

Living with Early Onset Dementia

ACKNOWLEDGMENTS

I wish to thank all those who care for me at this point of my journey. I would love to name a few that stick out of my memory and apologize to anyone I forget. Thank you, Adele, Nicole, Sherry and Lucretia (who is also family. And a special shout out to Karen for keeping my finances in order. My family for putting up with me and still managing to love me. My love to all of you. I might forget who you are, but my heart will always remember that I love you.

Living with Early Onset Dementia

CHAPTER 1: UNDERSTANDING EARLY ONSET DEMENTIA

Dementia is a general term that refers to a decline in cognitive function that is severe enough to interfere with daily activities. There are several different types of dementia, including Alzheimer's disease, vascular dementia, Lewy body dementia, and frontotemporal dementia. In this chapter, we will focus on early onset dementia, which is a type of dementia that affects people under the age of 65.

Early onset dementia is a rare form of the disease, accounting for only about 5% of all cases. However, it can be particularly devastating, as it often strikes people in the prime of their lives, when they are still working, raising children, and pursuing their passions. Early onset dementia can also be more difficult to diagnose, as doctors may be less likely to suspect dementia in younger patients and may attribute early symptoms to stress or other conditions.

The causes of early onset dementia are not yet fully understood, but researchers believe that a combination of genetic, environmental, and lifestyle factors may play a role. Some people may have a genetic predisposition to the disease, while others may develop it as a result of head injuries, infections, or other medical conditions. Lifestyle factors such as diet, exercise, and sleep may also affect the risk of developing dementia.

Symptoms of early onset dementia can vary, but often include memory loss, confusion, difficulty with language, changes in personality or behavior, and problems with executive function (such as planning and decision-making). These symptoms may develop gradually or may appear suddenly and may be more difficult to recognize in younger people who are still active and engaged in their daily lives.

If you or a loved one is experiencing symptoms of early onset dementia, it is important to seek medical attention right away. Early diagnosis and treatment can help to slow the progression of the disease and may improve quality of life for both the patient and their family. There are also many resources available to help people with dementia and their caregivers, including support groups, counseling, and respite care services.

In the next chapter, we will explore the different types of early onset dementia in more detail, including their causes, symptoms, and treatments. We will also discuss some of the latest scientific breakthroughs in the field of dementia research, and how they may one day lead to a cure for this devastating disease.

CHAPTER 2: TYPES OF EARLY ONSET DEMENTIA

Early onset dementia is a rare condition that affects people under the age of 65. While there are several different types of dementia, some types are more commonly associated with early onset than others. In this chapter, we will explore the different types of early onset dementia, including their causes, symptoms, and treatments.

1. Alzheimer's Disease Alzheimer's disease is the most common type of dementia, and it affects people of all ages. However, it is also one of the most common types of early onset dementia, accounting for around 50% of cases. Alzheimer's disease is characterized by the buildup of abnormal proteins in the brain, which cause damage to nerve cells and disrupt the normal functioning of the brain. Symptoms of Alzheimer's disease include memory loss, confusion, difficulty with language, and changes in mood or behavior.

2. Vascular Dementia Vascular dementia is the second most common type of dementia, and it is caused by a lack of blood flow to the brain. This can be due to a stroke or other blockages in the blood vessels that supply the brain.

Vascular dementia is more common in people who have high blood pressure, high cholesterol, or other risk factors for cardiovascular disease. Symptoms of vascular dementia can include memory loss, confusion, difficulty with speech, and problems with motor function.

3. Frontotemporal Dementia Frontotemporal dementia is a less common type of dementia that affects the frontal and temporal lobes of the brain. This type of dementia is often associated with changes in personality and behavior, such as a lack of empathy, social withdrawal, and inappropriate or compulsive behaviors. Symptoms of frontotemporal dementia may also include problems with language, memory, and motor function.

4. Lewy Body Dementia Lewy body dementia is a type of dementia that is caused by the buildup of abnormal proteins in the brain, similar to Alzheimer's disease. However, Lewy body dementia is characterized by the presence of Lewy bodies, which are abnormal protein deposits that can be found in nerve cells throughout the brain. Symptoms of Lewy body dementia can include memory loss, confusion, hallucinations, and problems with movement.

5. Mixed Dementia Mixed dementia is a combination of two or more types of dementia, often Alzheimer's disease and vascular dementia. This type of dementia is more common in older adults, but it can also affect people with early onset dementia. Symptoms of mixed dementia can include memory loss, confusion, difficulty with language and motor function, and changes in personality or behavior.

While there is currently no cure for early onset dementia, there are treatments and strategies that can help to manage symptoms and improve quality of life for patients and their families. In the next chapter, we will explore some of the latest breakthroughs in dementia research, including new treatments and potential cures for this devastating disease.

CHAPTER 3: ADVANCES IN EARLY ONSET DEMENTIA RESEARCH

Over the past decade, there have been significant advancements in our understanding of early onset dementia and its causes, as well as new treatments and potential cures for this devastating disease. In this chapter, we will explore some of the latest breakthroughs in early onset dementia research.

1. Genetics and Early Onset Dementia One of the most exciting areas of early onset dementia research is genetics. Studies have identified several genes that are associated with an increased risk of developing dementia, including the APOE gene, which is associated with Alzheimer's disease. More recently, researchers have identified several other genes that may play a role in early onset dementia, including the TREM2 gene, which is involved in the immune system's response to brain damage. By understanding the genetic factors that contribute to early onset dementia, researchers may be able to develop new therapies and treatments that target these specific genes.

2. Imaging and Early Detection Another area of early onset dementia research is the use of imaging techniques to detect the early signs of dementia. Magnetic resonance imaging (MRI) and positron emission tomography (PET) scans can provide detailed images of the brain and help to identify abnormalities that may be indicative of dementia. These imaging techniques are also being used to develop new drugs that can target specific areas of the brain and slow the progression of dementia.

3. Stem Cell Therapy Stem cell therapy is another promising area of early onset dementia research. Researchers are exploring the use of stem cells to replace damaged brain cells and restore cognitive function in patients with dementia. While this research is still in the early stages, initial results have been promising, and there is hope that stem cell therapy may one day be an effective treatment for early onset dementia.

4. Lifestyle Interventions Research has also shown that lifestyle interventions can be effective in reducing the risk of developing early onset dementia. Regular exercise, a healthy diet, and mental stimulation have all been shown to be effective in maintaining cognitive function and

reducing the risk of dementia. In addition, social engagement and a strong support network can also help to improve quality of life for patients with early onset dementia.

While there is still much work to be done, these breakthroughs in early onset dementia research provide hope for the millions of people who are affected by this devastating disease. By continuing to invest in research and development, we may one day be able to find a cure for early onset dementia and improve the lives of patients and their families.

CHAPTER 4: COPING STRATEGIES FOR EARLY ONSET DEMENTIA

Being diagnosed with early onset dementia can be devastating for both the individual and their loved ones. However, there are coping strategies that can help to manage the symptoms and improve quality of life. In this chapter, we will explore some of the most effective coping strategies for early onset dementia.

1. Education and Support One of the most important coping strategies for early onset dementia is education and support. It is important for the individual and their family members to understand the disease and its progression, as well as the available treatment options. Support groups and counseling services can also provide emotional support and guidance for both the individual and their loved ones.

2. Regular Exercise Regular exercise has been shown to be effective in maintaining cognitive function and improving overall health for individuals with early onset dementia. Physical activity can help to reduce stress and anxiety, improve mood, and enhance brain function.

3. Social Engagement Social engagement is also important for individuals with early onset dementia. Staying active and engaged with family members, friends, and community groups can help to improve mood and cognitive function and reduce the risk of depression and isolation.

4. Brain-Boosting Activities Engaging in brain-boosting activities such as reading, puzzles, and learning new skills can help to maintain cognitive function and delay the progression of early onset dementia. These activities can also provide a sense of accomplishment and improve self-esteem.

5. Adaptations to Daily Life As early onset dementia progresses, it may become necessary to make adaptations to daily life to help manage symptoms and maintain independence. This may include simplifying daily routines, using memory aids such as calendars and reminder systems, and modifying the living environment to reduce safety risks.

6. Medication and Therapy In addition to lifestyle interventions, medication and therapy can also be effective in managing the symptoms of early onset dementia. Medications such as

cholinesterase inhibitors and memantine can improve cognitive function, while therapy such as occupational and speech therapy can help to maintain independence and improve communication skills.

While there is no cure for early onset dementia, these coping strategies can help to manage symptoms and improve quality of life for individuals and their loved ones. By taking a proactive approach and seeking support and guidance, individuals with early onset dementia can continue to live fulfilling lives for as long as possible.

CHAPTER 5: COMMUNICATION STRATEGIES FOR EARLY ONSET DEMENTIA

One of the most challenging aspects of early onset dementia is communication. As the disease progresses, individuals may experience difficulty communicating their thoughts and feelings, and may become frustrated or withdrawn. In this chapter, we will explore some effective communication strategies for individuals with early onset dementia and their loved ones.

1. Maintain Eye Contact Maintaining eye contact can help to establish a connection and convey respect and understanding. Individuals with early onset dementia may become distracted or disoriented, so maintaining eye contact can help to focus their attention and promote clear communication.

2. Use Simple Language Using simple, clear language can help to minimize confusion and reduce frustration. Avoid using complex or abstract concepts and stick to simple, concrete language. Break down information into smaller, easier-to-understand pieces.

3. Use Visual Aids Visual aids such as pictures, drawings, and diagrams can help to convey information and make communication easier. Visual aids can also be used to provide cues and reminders, such as pictures of family members or items that are frequently used.

4. Use Non-Verbal Cues Non-verbal cues such as facial expressions, gestures, and body language can help to convey emotions and meaning when words are difficult to find. For example, a smile or a hug can convey love and affection even when words are difficult to express.

5. Encourage Expression Encouraging expression can help to promote communication and reduce frustration. Provide opportunities for the individual to express themselves through activities such as art, music, and writing.

6. Practice Active Listening Active listening involves fully focusing on the individual and being present in the moment. This can help to promote clear communication and reduce misunderstandings. Avoid interrupting and show that you are listening by nodding and acknowledging the individual's feelings.

7. Be Patient and Understanding Finally, it is important to be patient and understanding when communicating with individuals with

early onset dementia. Remember that they may become frustrated or confused and may need extra time and support to communicate effectively. Be empathetic and respectful, and provide support and guidance as needed.

By using these communication strategies, individuals with early onset dementia and their loved ones can continue to maintain meaningful connections and communicate effectively throughout the progression of the disease.

CHAPTER 6: LEGAL AND FINANCIAL PLANNING FOR EARLY ONSET DEMENTIA

Early onset dementia can have a significant impact on an individual's ability to manage their finances and make legal decisions. It is important for individuals with early onset dementia and their loved ones to plan ahead and make necessary legal and financial arrangements. In this chapter, we will explore some important considerations and strategies for legal and financial planning for early onset dementia.

1. Power of Attorney A power of attorney is a legal document that designates a trusted individual to make legal and financial decisions on behalf of the individual with early onset dementia. This can include managing bank accounts, paying bills, and making medical decisions. It is important to choose someone who is trustworthy and capable of managing these responsibilities.

2. Advance Directives Advance directives are legal documents that outline an individual's wishes

for medical care in the event that they become unable to make decisions for themselves. This can include preferences for life-sustaining treatment and end-of-life care. Advance directives can help to ensure that the individual's wishes are respected and can reduce stress and confusion for loved ones.

3. Financial Planning Financial planning is an important consideration for individuals with early onset dementia. It may be necessary to make arrangements for long-term care and manage finances to ensure that they are sufficient to cover medical expenses and other costs. This may include working with a financial advisor to create a budget and plan for retirement.

4. Estate Planning Estate planning involves making arrangements for the distribution of assets after an individual's death. This can include creating a will, establishing a trust, and designating beneficiaries for life insurance policies and retirement accounts. Estate planning can help to ensure that an individual's assets are distributed according to their wishes and can minimize stress and conflict for loved ones.

5. Guardianship and Conservatorship In some

cases, it may be necessary to establish guardianship or conservatorship for an individual with early onset dementia. This involves appointing a legal guardian or conservator to manage the individual's affairs and make decisions on their behalf. This can be a complex and emotional process, so it is important to seek guidance from an experienced attorney.

By taking proactive steps to plan for legal and financial issues, individuals with early onset dementia and their loved ones can reduce stress and uncertainty and ensure that their wishes are respected. Seeking guidance from legal and financial professionals can help to ensure that these arrangements are comprehensive and effective.

CHAPTER 7: MANAGING CHALLENGING BEHAVIORS IN EARLY ONSET DEMENTIA

Early onset dementia can cause changes in behavior and personality, which can be challenging for both the individual with dementia and their loved ones. In this chapter, we will explore some strategies for managing challenging behaviors in early onset dementia.

1. Identify Triggers One of the first steps in managing challenging behaviors is to identify triggers that may be causing the behavior. Common triggers may include environmental factors, such as noise or changes in routine, or physical factors, such as hunger or pain.

2. Create a Calm Environment Creating a calm and supportive environment can help to reduce stress and anxiety for individuals with early onset dementia. This may include minimizing noise and distractions, providing comfortable and familiar surroundings, and establishing a predictable routine.

3. Maintain a Structured Routine A structured routine can help to reduce confusion and provide a sense of security and stability for

individuals with early onset dementia. This may include establishing a regular schedule for meals, activities, and rest.

4. Use Positive Reinforcement Positive reinforcement can be an effective strategy for managing challenging behaviors. This involves rewarding positive behaviors with praise, attention, or tangible rewards, such as favorite foods or activities.

5. Avoid Arguing or Correcting Arguing or correcting the individual with dementia can often escalate challenging behaviors. Instead, it is important to remain calm and redirect the individual's attention to a more positive activity or topic.

6. Engage in Activities Engaging in activities can help to reduce boredom and provide a sense of purpose for individuals with early onset dementia. Activities can include hobbies, exercise, and socializing with friends and family.

7. Use Medications Carefully Medications can be an effective tool for managing challenging behaviors in early onset dementia, but they should be used carefully and under the guidance of a healthcare provider. Some medications may have side effects or

interactions with other medications, so it is important to closely monitor their use.

By using these strategies, individuals with early onset dementia and their loved ones can effectively manage challenging behaviors and maintain a supportive and positive environment. It is important to work closely with healthcare providers and other professionals to develop a comprehensive care plan that addresses the individual's unique needs and preferences.

CHAPTER 8: MAINTAINING QUALITY OF LIFE FOR INDIVIDUALS WITH EARLY ONSET DEMENTIA

Early onset dementia can have a significant impact on an individual's quality of life, as it can affect their ability to perform daily activities and participate in social and recreational activities. In this chapter, we will explore some strategies for maintaining quality of life for individuals with early onset dementia.

1. Focus on Abilities While dementia can cause changes in cognitive function and physical abilities, it is important to focus on the individual's remaining abilities and strengths. This may include adapting activities or tasks to match their abilities and providing opportunities for success and engagement.

2. Engage in Meaningful Activities Engaging in meaningful activities can help to maintain a sense of purpose and identity for individuals with early onset dementia. This may include hobbies, volunteering, and spending time with friends and family.

3. Provide Opportunities for Socialization

Socialization is an important aspect of maintaining quality of life for individuals with early onset dementia. This may include participating in group activities, attending social events, and spending time with family and friends.

4. Promote Physical Activity Physical activity can help to maintain physical health and promote a sense of well-being for individuals with early onset dementia. This may include activities such as walking, swimming, or participating in low-impact exercise programs.

5. Use Technology to Enhance Engagement Technology can be a useful tool for enhancing engagement and quality of life for individuals with early onset dementia. This may include using virtual reality programs, digital games, or online communication platforms to connect with others and engage in meaningful activities.

6. Provide Support for Caregivers Maintaining quality of life for individuals with early onset dementia also involves providing support for caregivers. This may include respite care, counseling, and educational resources to help caregivers manage the demands of caregiving and maintain their own well-being.

By focusing on abilities, engaging in meaningful activities, providing opportunities for socialization and physical activity, using technology, and supporting caregivers, individuals with early onset dementia can maintain a high quality of life and continue to participate in activities that bring them joy and fulfillment. It is important to work closely with healthcare providers and other professionals to develop a care plan that addresses the individual's unique needs and preferences.

CHAPTER 9: COMMUNICATION STRATEGIES FOR EARLY ONSET DEMENTIA

Early onset dementia can cause changes in communication abilities, making it difficult for individuals with dementia to express themselves and interact with others. In this chapter, we will explore some communication strategies for individuals with early onset dementia.

1. Use Clear and Simple Language Using clear and simple language can help individuals with early onset dementia better understand and respond to communication. This may involve using short sentences, avoiding complex or abstract concepts, and speaking slowly and clearly.

2. Be Patient and Supportive It is important to be patient and supportive when communicating with individuals with early onset dementia. This may involve allowing extra time for them to process information and respond, using visual aids or gestures to enhance understanding, and offering reassurance and validation.

3. Listen Actively Active listening involves paying attention to the individual's verbal and nonverbal cues and responding with empathy and understanding. This may involve using

reflective listening techniques, such as summarizing or paraphrasing the individual's statements, to ensure that you have accurately understood their message.

4. Use Nonverbal Communication Nonverbal communication, such as facial expressions, gestures, and tone of voice, can be an effective tool for communicating with individuals with early onset dementia. This may involve using a warm and friendly tone of voice, maintaining eye contact, and using physical touch or gestures to convey emotions or reinforce messages.

5. Avoid Overstimulation Individuals with early onset dementia may become easily overwhelmed or overstimulated by environmental factors, such as noise or bright lights. It is important to avoid overstimulation and create a calm and supportive environment for communication.

6. Adapt Communication to the Individual's Needs Communication strategies may need to be adapted to meet the individual's unique needs and preferences. This may involve using assistive technologies, such as communication boards or speech-generating devices, or adapting communication styles to match the

individual's cultural or linguistic background.

By using these communication strategies, individuals with early onset dementia can continue to communicate effectively and maintain connections with their loved ones and caregivers. It is important to work closely with healthcare providers and other professionals to develop a comprehensive care plan that addresses the individual's unique communication needs and preferences.

CHAPTER 10: CONCLUSION

Early onset dementia is a challenging diagnosis that can have a significant impact on individuals and their families. However, with early detection and appropriate care and support, individuals with early onset dementia can continue to live meaningful and fulfilling lives.

In this book, we have explored the various forms of dementia, including Alzheimer's disease, vascular dementia, frontotemporal dementia, and Lewy body dementia. We have also discussed the latest scientific breakthroughs and advancements in the diagnosis and treatment of dementia.

Furthermore, we have examined strategies for managing the symptoms of early onset dementia, including medication, lifestyle changes, and alternative therapies. We have also explored ways to maintain quality of life and promote effective communication for individuals with early onset dementia.

Overall, this book aims to provide a

comprehensive overview of early onset dementia and empower individuals and their caregivers to take an active role in managing the condition. By working closely with healthcare providers, developing a care plan, and utilizing appropriate resources and support, individuals with early onset dementia can continue to live fulfilling lives and maintain connections with their loved ones.

ABOUT THE AUTHOR

My name is Lisa Head and I taught music for many years at public school in Indiana for 28 years. Lived near Plymouth, IN all that time. The schools I taught at were LaVille JR-SR and at LaVille Elementary. I am the proud mom of three young men, Aiden, Randy and Jesse. They have definitely helped me to stay alert and on my toes. Love them with all my heart. I wrote this book with the help of AI Chat. I gave the directions, but AI wrote this book, I just to formate it. It is a blessing that is helping me educate people about dementia. Thank you for taking the time to read it!

www.ingramcontent.com/pod-product-compliance
Lightning Source LLC
Chambersburg PA
CBHW071121220526
45467CB00004B/2001